Once upon a time in homes much like your own, families were beginning to become aware of the many toxins and chemicals that were invading their everyday lives. The products that touched their skin, the air they breathed, even the foods they ate were loaded with junk, so they began to do a little research. A kind friend opened their eyes to a whole new world of natural products they could feel good about using on and around their children. This information is too good not to share with you too!

Follow along as we journey through some of those simple Young Living products that may just change the way you look at the products you purchase and apply to yourself and your children on a daily basis.

KIDSCENTS® MAKES SENSE

If you are looking for an easy way to start using essential oils with your children, KidScents® makes sense and takes the guess work out of which oils to use and how to properly dilute. These mild and gentle blends come pre-diluted with coconut oil and are perfect for children 2-12 years old. Diffuse a few drops of GeneYus™ to keep young minds focused and on task during homework hour. With the outdoors, often come unplanned bumps in the road. Apply a roller ball fitment and keep Owie™ in your purse for those "owie" moments. SleepyIze™ contains oils that are great for diffusing or applying topically at bedtime. The name SniffleEase™ says it all with this refreshing blend. TummyGize™ is another blend you will feel good about keeping a roller ball fitment on top of to hand to your child to apply topically to their belly before or after meal time.

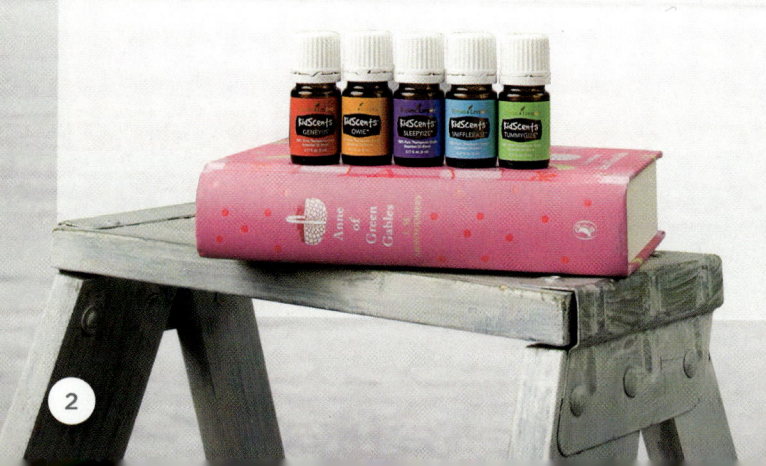

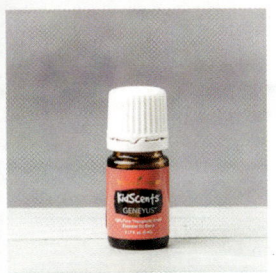

GENEYUS™

- Blend of Coconut oil, Sacred Frankincense, Blue Cypress, Cedarwood, Idaho Blue Spruce, Palo Santo, Melissa, Northern Lights Black spruce, Sweet Almond Oil, Bergamot, Myrrh, Vetiver, Geranium, Royal Hawaiian Sandalwood, Ylang ylang, Hyssop, Coriander, and Rose essential oils
- GeneYus™ is an excellent blend to diffuse, for young minds that are focusing and concentrating on projects

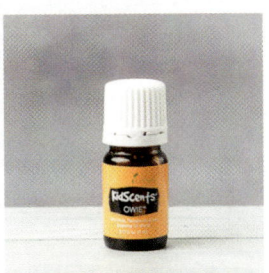

OWIE™

- Blend of Coconut oil, Idaho Balsam Fir, Tea tree, Helichrysum, Elemi, Cistus, Hinoki, and Clove essential oils
- Apply Owie™ topically to improve the appearance of your child's skin

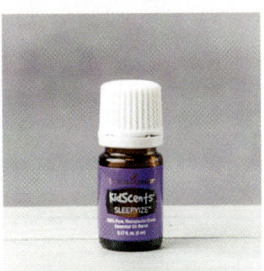

SLEEPYIZE™

- Blend of Coconut oil, Lavender, Geranium, Roman Chamomile, Tangerine, Bergamot, Sacred Frankincense, Valerian, and Rue essential oils
- Diffuse SleepyIze™ at bedtime for a peaceful aromatic environment

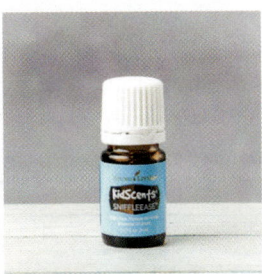

SNIFFLEEASE™

- Blend of Coconut oil, Eucalyptus Blue, Palo Santo, Lavender, Dorado Azul, Ravintsara, Myrtle, Eucalyptus Globulus, Marjoram, Pine, Eucalyptus Citriodora, Cypress, Eucalyptus Radiata, Black Spruce, and Peppermint essential oils
- SniffleEase™ is a rejuvenating and refreshing blend formulated just for kids

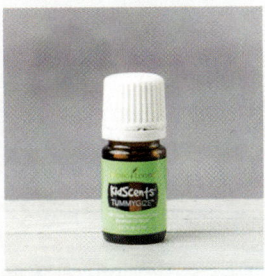

TUMMYGIZE™

- Blend of Coconut oil, Spearmint, Peppermint, Tangerine, Fennel, Anise, Ginger, and Cardamom essential oils
- TummyGize™ is a relaxing, quieting blend that can be applied to little tummies

YOU'RE NEVER FULLY DRESSED WITHOUT A SMILE

One of the first & obvious places to begin removing toxins from your child's life is on the bathroom counters. Your kids will love using these gentle and effective products! Thieves Foaming Hand Soap makes it easy to lather, rinse, and get on your way! With a plant-based, instant-foam formula, skin is left feeling clean, refreshed, and never over-dried. The Slique™ Toothpaste is a safe and effective blend that promotes healthy teeth without the use of fluoride, dyes, synthetic colors, artificial flavors, or preservatives. Your big kids will enjoy having fresh breath and a pleasant taste with the Thieves Mouthwash to give them the confidence to face their day ahead.

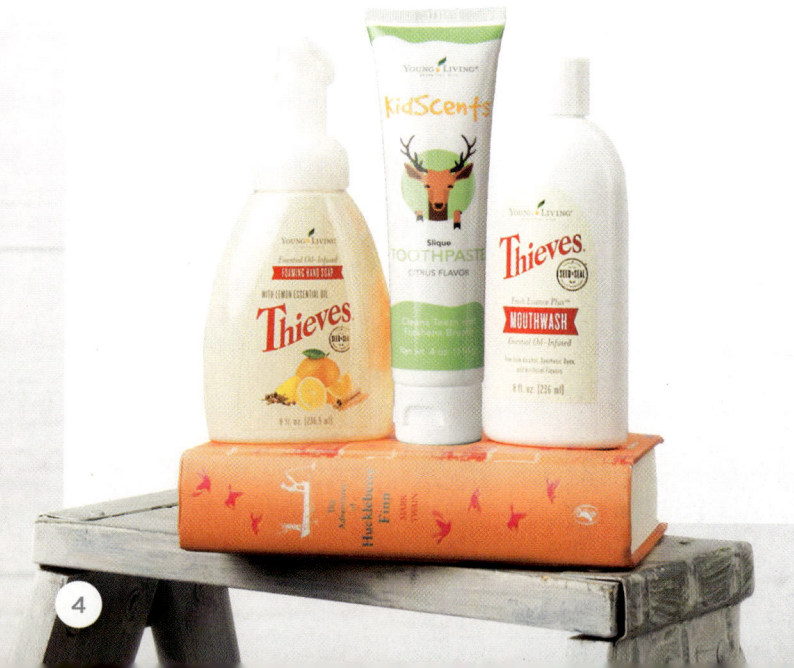

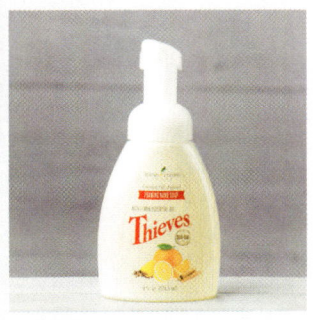

THIEVES® FOAMING HAND SOAP

- Combines Thieves blend, Lemon and Orange essential oils with other naturally derived ingredients to clean hands
- Instant foam makes it easy to lather and rinse
- Contains no sulfates, dyes, synthetic fragrances, or harsh chemicals

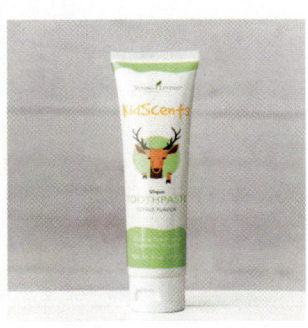

KIDSCENTS® SLIQUE™ TOOTHPASTE

- Use morning, night, and after meals to help young smiles stay healthy and vibrant
- Contains no fluoride, dyes, synthetic colors, artificial flavors, or preservatives

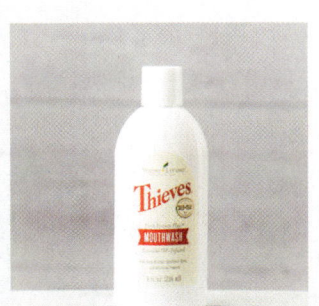

THIEVES® MOUTHWASH

- Supports healthy-looking gums and teeth
- Provides a refreshing taste with 100 percent pure essential oils
- Contains no alcohol, dyes, or artificial flavors

RUB, A DUB, DUB FUN IN THE TUB

If the products you are using to wash and clean your child's skin are rainbow colored, and smell like birthday cake, you may want to research those ingredients before it's time for the next bath. Create your own bubble bath with the KidScents® Bath Gel. Formulated with natural MSM, aloe vera, antioxidants, and pure Lemon & Cedarwood essential oils, this liquid soap is pH balanced for children's skin. The KidScents® Shampoo pleasantly scented with Chamomile, Tangerine, and Lemon essential oils effectively and gently cleanse without irritating your children's skin.

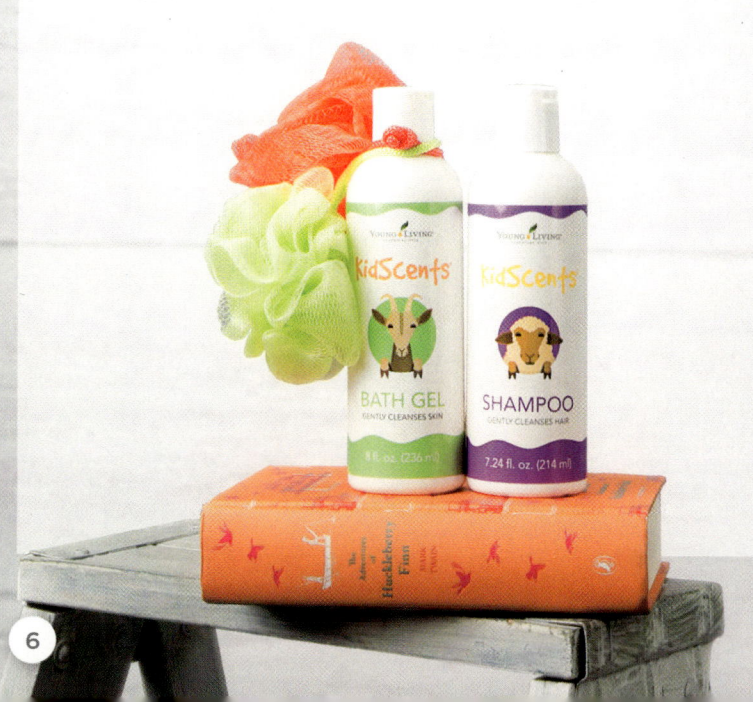

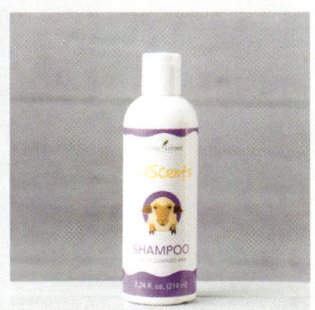

KIDSCENTS® SHAMPOO

- Effectively and gently cleanses without causing irritation
- No mineral oils, synthetic perfumes, artificial colorings, or toxic ingredients

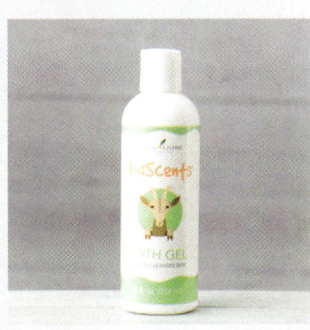

KIDSCENTS® BATH GEL

- Safe, gentle soap that cleanses and protects sensitive skin
- pH balanced for children's skin
- No mineral oils, synthetic perfumes, artificial colorings, or toxic ingredients

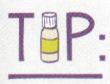

TIP: Try adding a few drops of Tea Tree essential oil to your child's shampoo to kick it up a notch.

ROLL, ROLL, ROLL IT ON

Many mothers have started creating their own DIY roller bottle blends in fancy bottles with labels found on various cute shops on the world wide web. A little secret you may not know about, Young Living has taken the "Stress Away" out of mixing up your own, by creating these ready made blends that are diluted with coconut oil. Even the smallest hands can rub a dab of Tranquil on their feet before bed, or glide Breathe Again across their chest for comfort during the winter months. You can breathe a sigh of Deep Relief reaching for these safe and effective products.

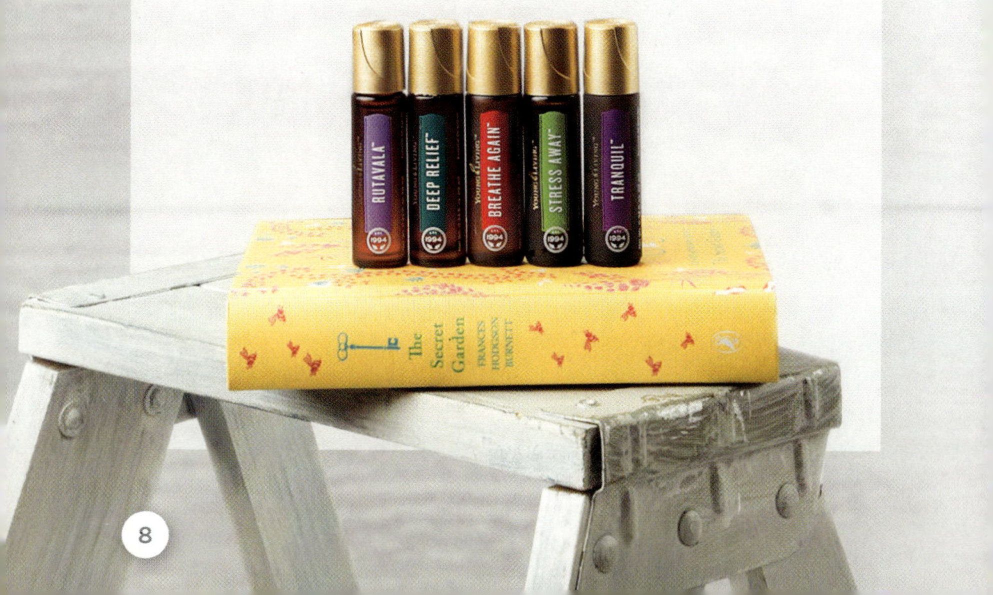

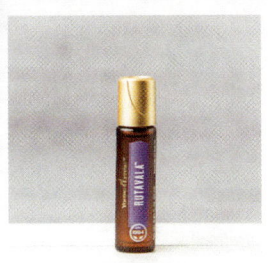

RUTAVALA™

- Blend of Coconut oil, Ruta, Valerian, and Lavender essential oils
- Apply to child's feet or wrists as part of a relaxing routine before bedtime
- Moms and Dads can enjoy the calming aroma before bedtime as well

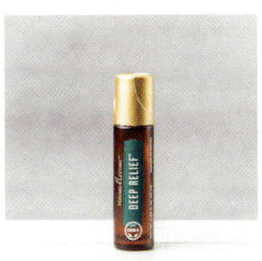

DEEP RELIEF™

- Blend of Coconut oil, Peppermint, Lemon, Canada Balsam, Clove, Balsam Copaiba, Wintergreen, Helichrysum, Vetiver, and Dorado Azul essential oils
- Provides a refreshing and cooling sensation for Mom after a workout or lifting and keeping up with children all day

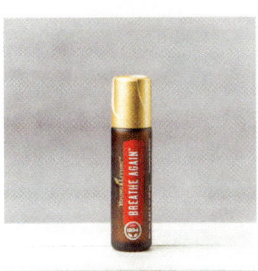

BREATHE AGAIN™

- Blend of Coconut oil, Eucalyptus Globulus, Laurus Nobilis, Rose Hip Oil, Peppermint, Eucalyptus Radiata, Balsam Copaiba, Blue Cypress, and Myrtle essential oils
- Jump Start your child's school day by applying the rejuvenating scent to their chest or under their nose

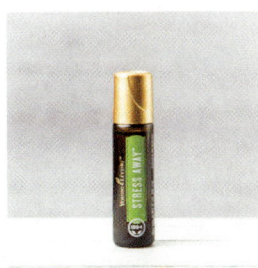

STRESS AWAY™

- Blend of Copaiba, Lime, Cedarwood, Vanilla, Ocotea, and Lavender essential oils
- Send kids to school on test day with Stress Away's soothing aroma
- Grab and go in purse or diaper bag when shopping with children

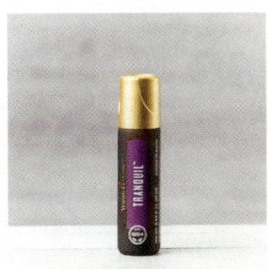

TRANQUIL™

- Blend of Coconut oil, Lavender, Cedarwood, and Roman Chamomile essential oils
- Kids can apply to the bottoms of their feet for a soothing bedtime routine
- Roll Tranquil over child's heart during troubling times for a centering aroma

I'M A BIG KID NOW

Growing children don't always get all the necessary nutrients from the foods they eat, so moms turn to vitamin supplements to help fill in some of the gaps. You can bypass many of the conventional sources that add hidden fillers and sugars. The MightyVites™ chewable tablets are a tasty, effective way to provide children the full spectrum of vitamins, minerals, antioxidants, and phytonutrients that are necessary for healthy development. Add a MightyZyme™ to help children combat the negative effects of enzyme depletion and address each of the digestive needs of growing bodies.

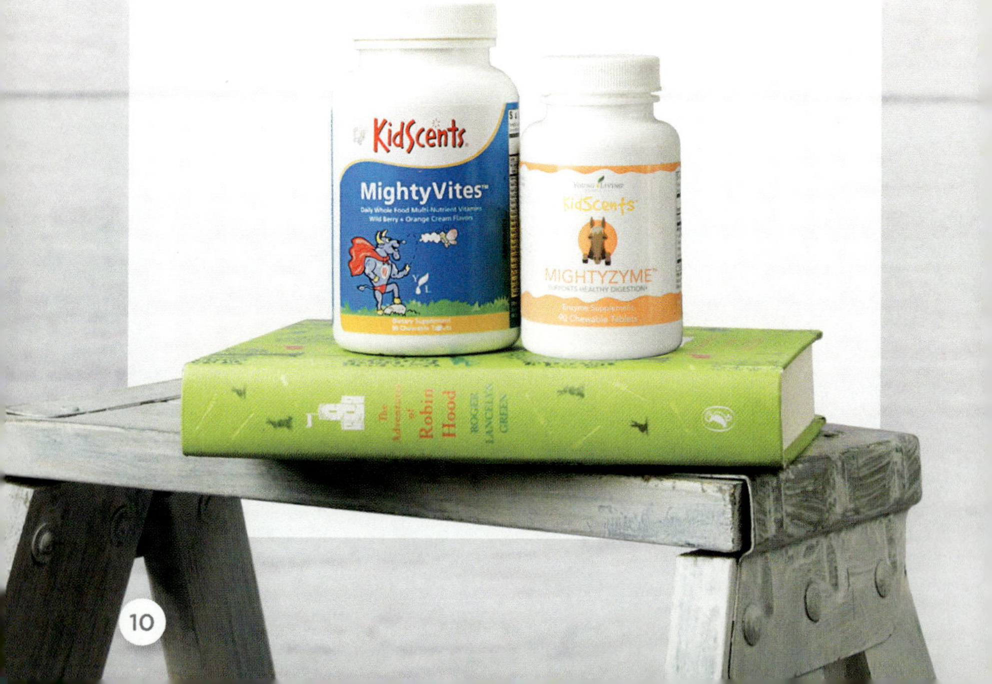

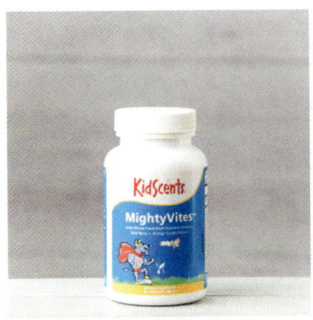

MIGHTYVITES™

- Children age 4-12 years old, take 3 tablets daily
- Contains Vitamin A, C, D, E, K, B1, B2, B3, B6, Folate, B12, Biotin, Panthothenic acid, Iodine, Magnesium, Zinc, Selenium, Copper, Chromium, Choline

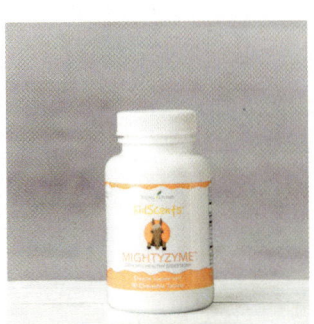

MIGHTYZYME™

- Take 3 times daily prior to or with meals
- For relief of occasional symptoms including fullness, pressure, bloating, stuffed feeling that may occur after eating

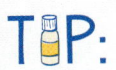

The KidScents® vitamins are chewable tablets that have a pleasing flavor for kids. Parents have also been known to open some of the Young Living supplement capsules and empty the contents into yogurt or other soft food for their children to get the vital nutrients without having to swallow a capsule. Multigreens, a nutritious chlorophyll formula, and the probiotic Life 9 are both excellent supplements with easy open capsules for all members of your family.

MAY I HAVE YOUR ATTENTION PLEASE

Have you ever told your child to complete a task one minute, and then the next minute they are off in a different direction and can't remember what you said? We all want to see our children excel and be able to stay focused on their childhood tasks and school work, so they can become productive adults. Equip your child with their own bottle of KidScents® GeneYus™ essential oil blend. Diffuse Peppermint, Citrus Fresh™, and Clarity™ together or separate for a happy homework hour. Try applying Frankincense topically to the base of the neck or behind ears to promote focus and attention; you might also try Young Living's Sacred Frankincense™ applied topically or diffused.

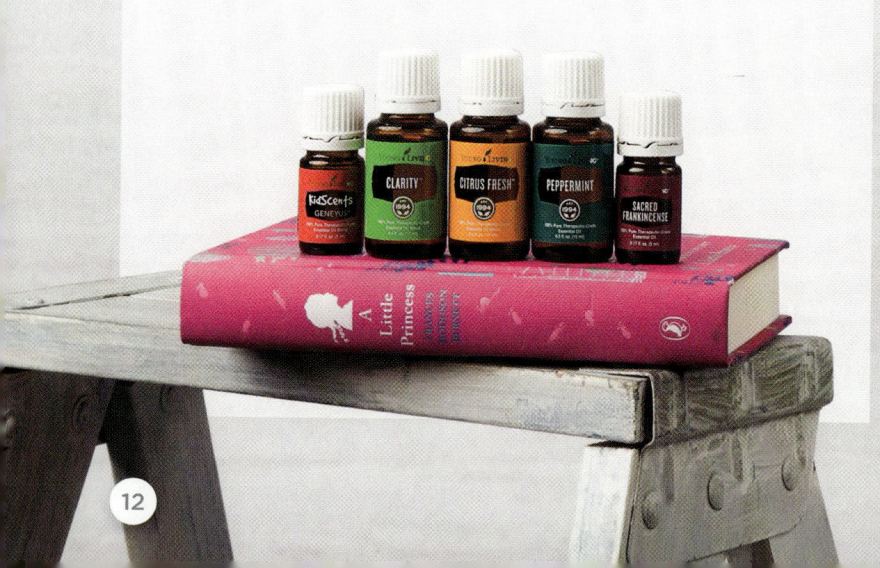

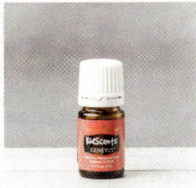

GENEYUS™

- Blend of Coconut oil, Sacred Frankincense, Blue Cypress, Cedarwood, Idaho Blue Spruce, Palo Santo, Melissa, Northern Lights Black Spruce, Sweet Almond Oil, Bergamot, Myrrh, Vetiver, Geranium, Royal Hawaiian Sandalwood, Ylang Ylang, Hyssop, Coriander, and Rose essential oils

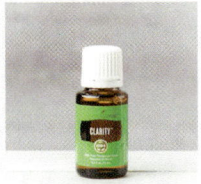

CLARITY™

- Blend of Basil, Cardamom, Rosemary, Peppermint, Coriander, Geranium, Bergamot, Lemon, Ylang Ylang, Jasmine, Roman Chamomile, and Palmarosa essential oils
- Apply a drop behind your child's ear before study time

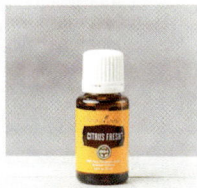

CITRUS FRESH™

- Blend of Orange, Tangerine, Grapefruit, Lemon, Mandarin, and Spearmint essential oils
- Diffuse in classrooms to help promote an aroma of positivity and creativity

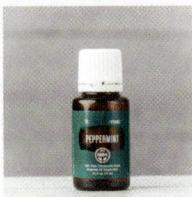

PEPPERMINT

- Add 10 drops to a roller bottle with a carrier oil for an "Up & At Em" roller blend
- Diffuse during testing, to help young minds focus

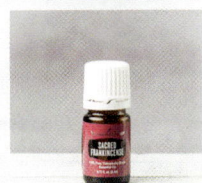

SACRED FRANKINCENSE™

- Diffuse in the morning hours to help attitudes and minds get focused for the day
- Add a drop to a diffuser necklace for a scented focus reminder throughout the day

AROMATIC PLAYDOUGH

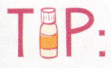
TIP:

- 2 cups flour
- 1/2 cup salt
- 2 tablespoons cream of tarter
- 2 tablespoons vegetable oil
- 10 drops essential oil (Citrus Fresh, Peppermint, Orange)
- 1.5 cups boiling water
- food coloring optional

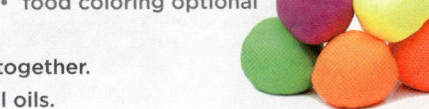

1. Mix flour, salt, and cream of tarter together.
2. Blend in vegetable oil and essential oils.
3. Stir in boiling water and knead dough with hands until moldable.
4. Add food coloring if color is desired.

1 SNACK, 2 SNACK
MY PACK, YOUR PACK

Have you ever stopped to consider how much sugar and artificial flavorings are in the pouches of juice that children consume as a matter of convenience? Why not invest in natural real energy for your child that will support overall wellness? NingXia Red® is a sweet and tangy powerhouse blend of wolfberry, plum, aronia, cherry, blueberry, and pomegranate juices and extracts, along with Lemon, Orange, Yuzu, and Tangerine essential oils. Pop packets in lunch boxes, traveling on the go, or freeze pouches for the perfect afternoon slushie popsicle. As one of the most amazing antioxidant drinks on the planet, you will want your whole family to enjoy this super food drink regularly.

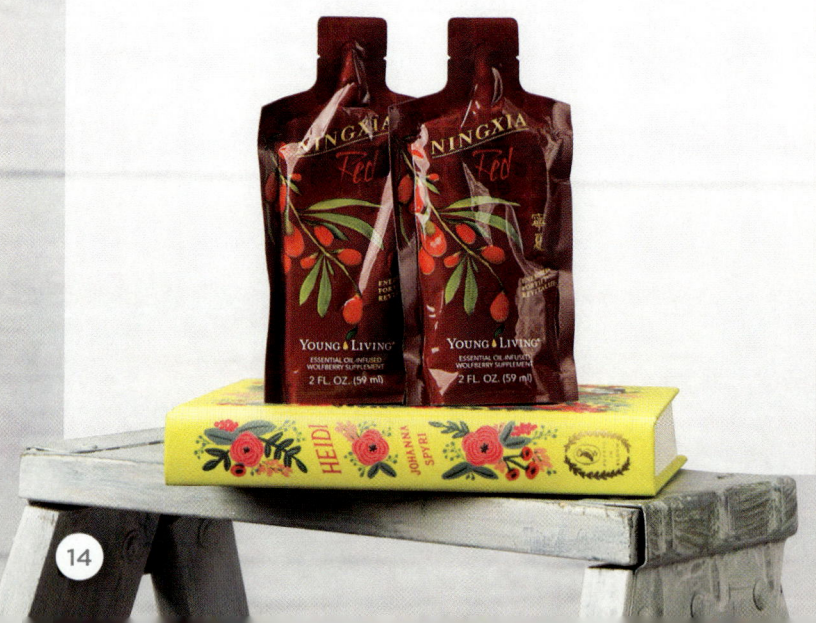

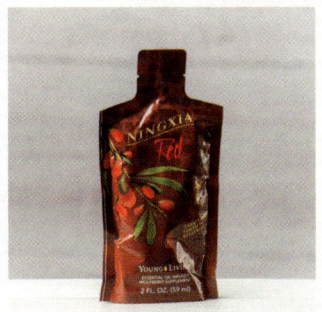

NINGXIA RED® SINGLES

- Convenient, portable pouches to keep anywhere you need it
- Pack NingXia Red singles in lunch boxes for your kids
- Best served chilled

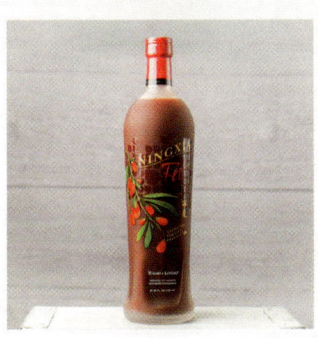

NINGXIA RED®

- Blend NingXia Red into a smoothie, acai bowl, or morning juice as part of a quick, convenient breakfast
- 4 ounces equals one serving of fruit

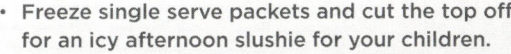

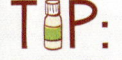 **TIP:**

- Freeze single serve packets and cut the top off for an icy afternoon slushie for your children.
- Mix NingXia Red with organic fruit juices and freeze in popsicle molds.
- Add a drop of Lemon or Orange Vitality for a sweet, zesty addition to your child's morning shot of NingXia.

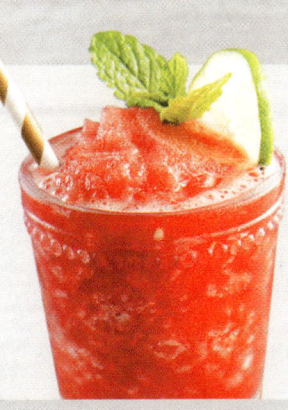

STOCK IT IN YOUR POCKET

Are your children being squirted with "antibacterial" gel everywhere they turn? Have you done any of your own research on this topic? Triclosan, alcohols, fragrances, to name a few, are known hormone disruptors. Give your children a voice and a choice to cleanse and purify their hands with Thieves® Waterless Hand Purifier. Kick it up a notch and safely spray ALL the many surfaces with the Thieves Spray that your children come in contact with. Yes, naturally derived plant-based ingredients, can be just as effective as chemical laden products. Polish off your pocket protection with a convenient moisturizing Lavender Lip Balm. You will want to make sure you are stocked with these three items before leaving the house!

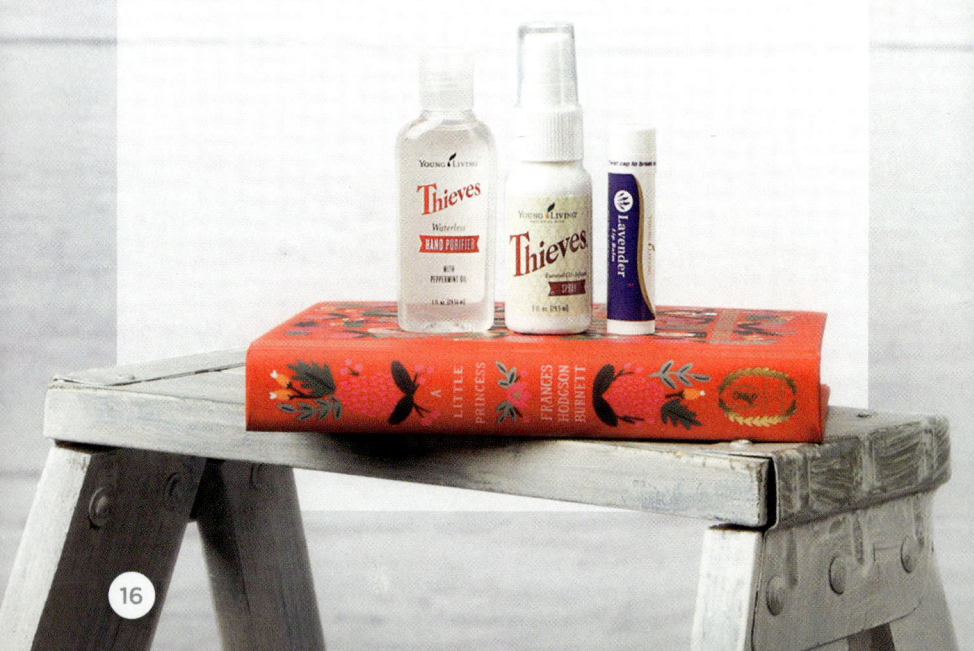

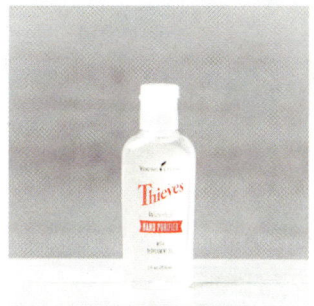

THIEVES® WATERLESS HAND PURIFIER

- Use daily as often as needed to clean hands
- Contains Peppermint essential oil
- Pack in purses and lunch boxes to purify hands before meals

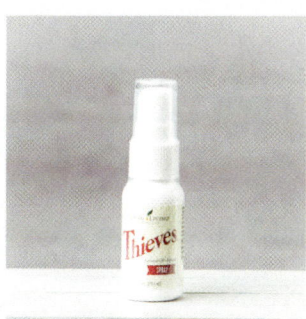

THIEVES® SPRAY

- Spray on light switches, sinks, door knobs, shopping carts, public bathrooms, counters, etc.
- Spray children's hands before meals
- Convenient size for pockets, purses, backpacks, & diaper bags

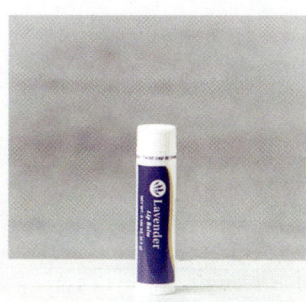

LAVENDER LIP BALM

- Nourish and moisturize little lips
- Perfect size to keep in pockets, backpacks, purses, & diaper bags
- Contains Coconut oil, Bees wax, Jojoba oil, Sweet Almond oil, Wolfberry seed oil, Rosehip seed oil, Vitamin E, and Lavender

FORGET COUNTING SHEEP

A restful night's sleep will make a difference in a child's mood and ability to focus and concentrate the next day. Help signal that it's bedtime with a nightly routine that gently transitions into quiet, peaceful rest. Create a calming and peaceful environment for your child by adding Lavender essential oil to a bath or diffuse during story time. Let your child pick the "sleepy" scent they like best, and even allow them to place a drop of SleepyIze™ on their wrist or roll Tranquil or RutaVaLa on the bottom of their feet. You may choose to share a few drops of the coveted Peace & Calming® blend in a diffuser in the kid's room, if you don't keep that one all to yourself.

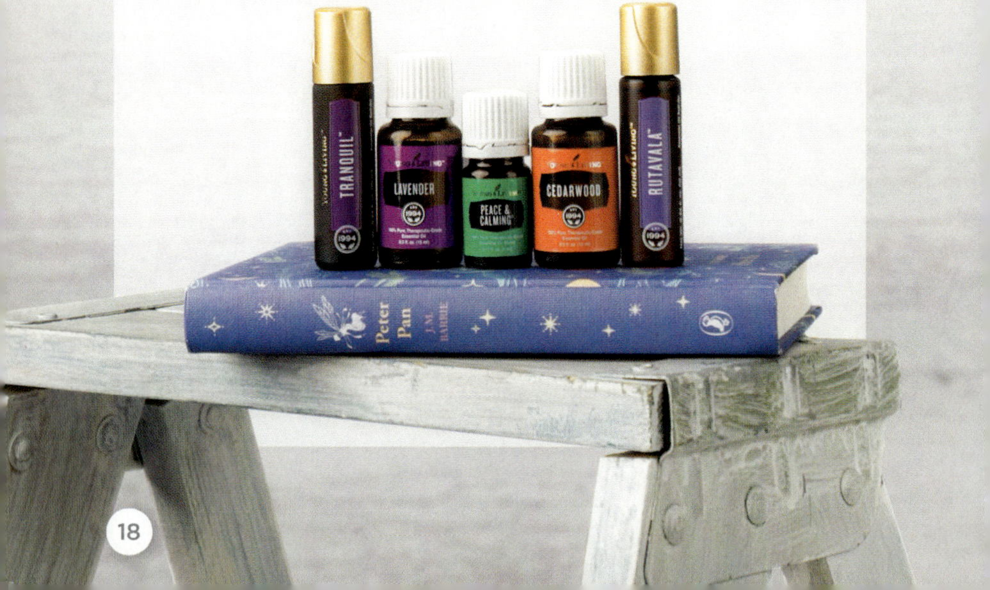

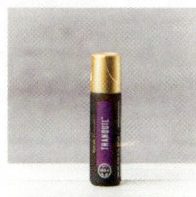

TRANQUIL™

- Blend of Coconut oil, Lavender, Cedarwood, and Roman Chamomile
- Apply to your child's feet or wrists as part of a relaxing routine before bedtime

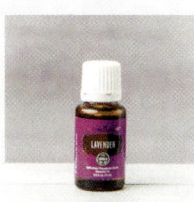

LAVENDER

- Rub oil on the bottom of your child's feet before bed or spritz pillows with distilled water and Lavender mixed in a spray bottle
- Add 3 drops to Epsom salts and add to your child's night time bath

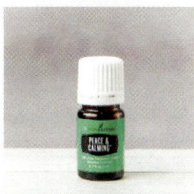

PEACE & CALMING®

- Blend of Tangerine, Orange, Ylang Ylang, Patchouli and Blue Tansy essential oils
- Add 2 drops to coconut oil and massage your child's back before nap time

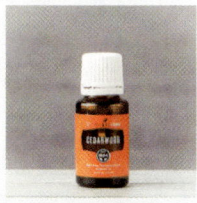

CEDARWOOD

- Pamper your child's hair with a drop in your child's shampoo
- Add 4 drops to a diffuser in your child's room at night

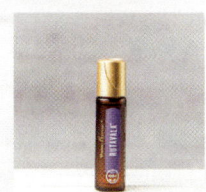

RUTAVALA™

- Blend of Coconut oil, Ruta, Valerian, and Lavender essential oils
- Apply to your child's feet or wrists as part of a relaxing routine before bedtime

SWEET DREAMS CREAM

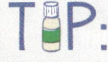

- 1/4 cup glass jar
- 5 drops Lavender
- 5 drops Peace & Calming
- 5 drops Cedarwood
- 1/4 cup coconut oil

Mix 1/4 cup coconut oil with drops of essential oils. Stir together well and store in a cool location with a secure lid. If cream becomes soft in warm weather, place in fridge to harden. Apply cream to bottoms of feet before going to bed.

ENJOY PLAYING IN THE GREAT OUTDOORS

We all want to enjoy the outdoors with our children. Without some sort of protection there is a price to be paid for long exposure to the sun and the pests that also enjoy the places we visit. Look up the effects of Oxybenzone found in many sunscreens and DEET found in many insect repellents. A little research will reveal products that are designed to keep us safe, often do more harm. Young Living's Mineral Sunscreen protects against UVA and UVB rays, providing 10 SPF with plant and mineral ingredients including non-nano zinc oxide. The insect repellent is formulated with a sesame seed base and infused with essential oils of Citronella, Lemongrass, Rosemary, Spearmint, Thyme and Clove for a pleasant topical application. The LavaDerm™ After-Sun Spray offers temporary relief from the pain and itching of minor burns, minor cuts, sunburns, scrapes, insect bites, and minor skin irritations, so your family can enjoy the great outdoors all day.

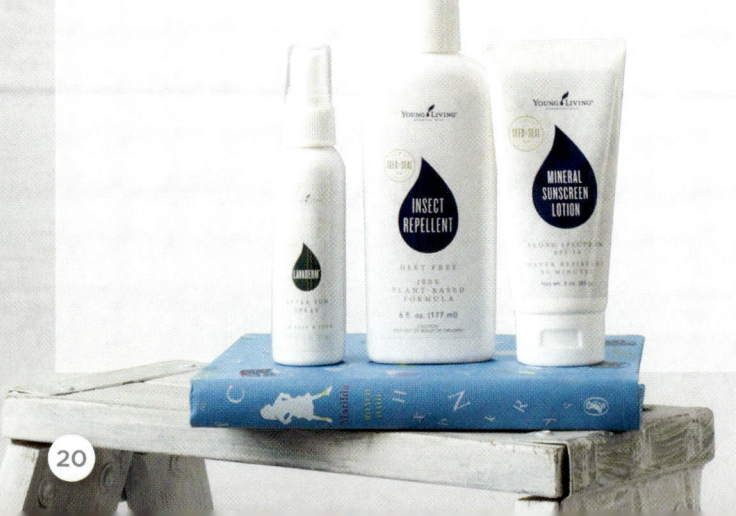

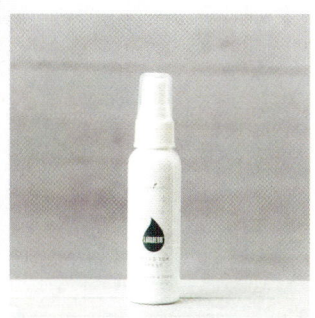

LAVADERM™ AFTER-SUN SPRAY

- Provides immediate relief
- Formulated without alcohol, parabens, phthalates, petrochemicals, animal-derived ingredients, synthetic preservatives, synthetic fragrances, or synthetic colorants

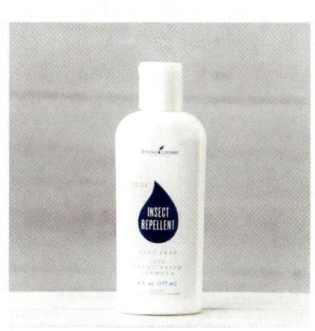

INSECT REPELLENT

- Clinically proven to repel mosquitoes and prevent bug bites
- Rubs easily into skin without a greasy or sticky finish
- Pure, gentle formula free from harsh chemicals and good for kids

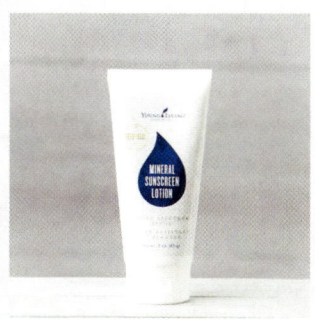

MINERAL SUNSCREEN LOTION

- Water and sweat resistant for 80 minutes
- Smooths easily onto skin and won't leave a white residue
- Contains essential oils of Helichrysum, Frankincense, & Carrot Seed

I THINK I CAN, I THINK I CAN

As humans, we often need a word of encouragement to keep a positive outlook. Situations in life can often seem scary, or we feel unprepared to face the tasks in front of us. Did you know when you smell an essential oil, the tiny molecules in the oil travel to the limbic system of the brain to change emotional thoughts? Give your children the boost of confidence they need to face speaking up in class, making new friends, and learning a new skill. You may try rubbing a drop of Valor™ on your child's wrists in the morning, or adding a drop to a diffuser necklace, so that the grounding scent can be accessed all day long. The earthy aroma of Vetiver can encourage feelings of positive self-reflection. Help your child Envision the GeneYus™ that is within themselves.

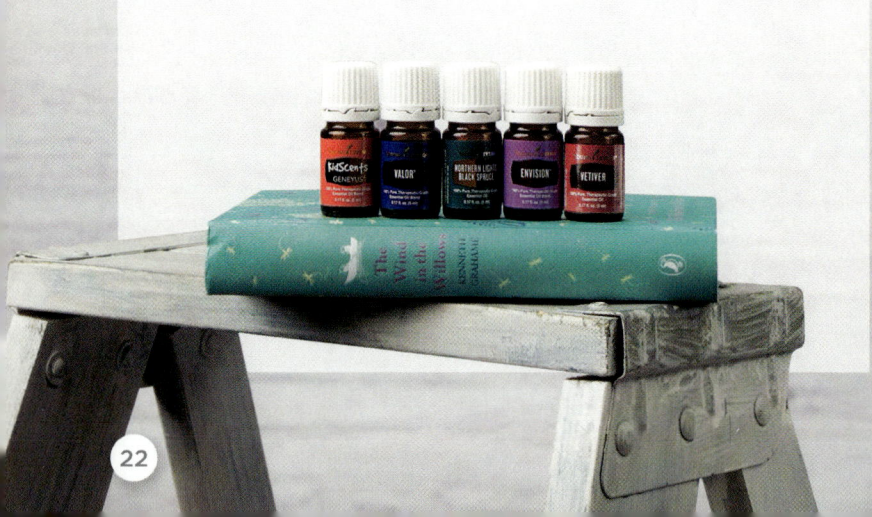

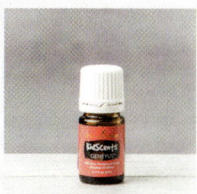

GENEYUS™

- Blend of Coconut oil, Sacred Frankincense, Blue Cypress, Cedarwood, Idaho Blue Spruce, Palo Santo, Melissa, Northern Lights Black Spruce, Sweet Almond Oil, Bergamot, Myrrh, Vetiver, Geranium, Royal Hawaiian Sandalwood, Ylang Ylang, Hyssop, Coriander, and Rose essential oils

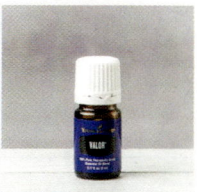

VALOR™

- Blend of Black Spruce, Camphor, Blue Tansy, Frankincense, and Geranium essential oils
- Mix a drop with coconut oil and massage into your child's neck and wrists before school

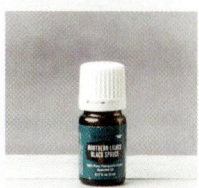

NORTHERN LIGHTS BLACK SPRUCE

- Add a drop to a diffuser bracelet for a boost of confidence to make new friends
- Diffuse in the afternoons for a grounding, fresh aromatic atmosphere

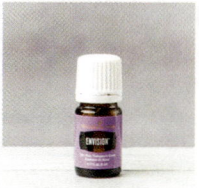

ENVISION™

- Blend of Black Spruce, Geranium, Orange, Lavender, Sage, and Rose essential oils
- Diffuse to stimulate feelings of creativity and resourcefulness to achieve childhood dreams

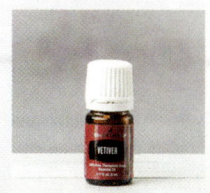

VETIVER

- Add a drop to a diffuser necklace for your child
- Combine equal parts of Vetiver, Cedarwood and Lavender with a carrier oil in a roller bottle for a great "Can Do" blend

DIFFUSER JEWELRY

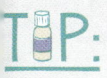 Children love having their own personal diffuser jewelry to wear their favorite empowering essential oil throughout the day. Girls will love a variety of locket necklaces that have felt pads inside to which you can add a drop of oil. Boys may enjoy having a leather cuff bracelet that they can add their favorite oil to.

THE NOSE KNOWS A GOOD THING

Once you begin diffusing essential oils in your home, you will quickly fall in love with the idea of having a diffuser in each room in your house! Of course your children will be over the moon excited when you can adorn their room or bathroom with the Dolphin Reef or Dino Land kids diffusers. The decorative cover is removable to add water and essential oils. Your children will long to fall asleep with their favorite calming essential oil and the 6 LED light choices. Your kids will love helping you make these kid approved diffuser blends!

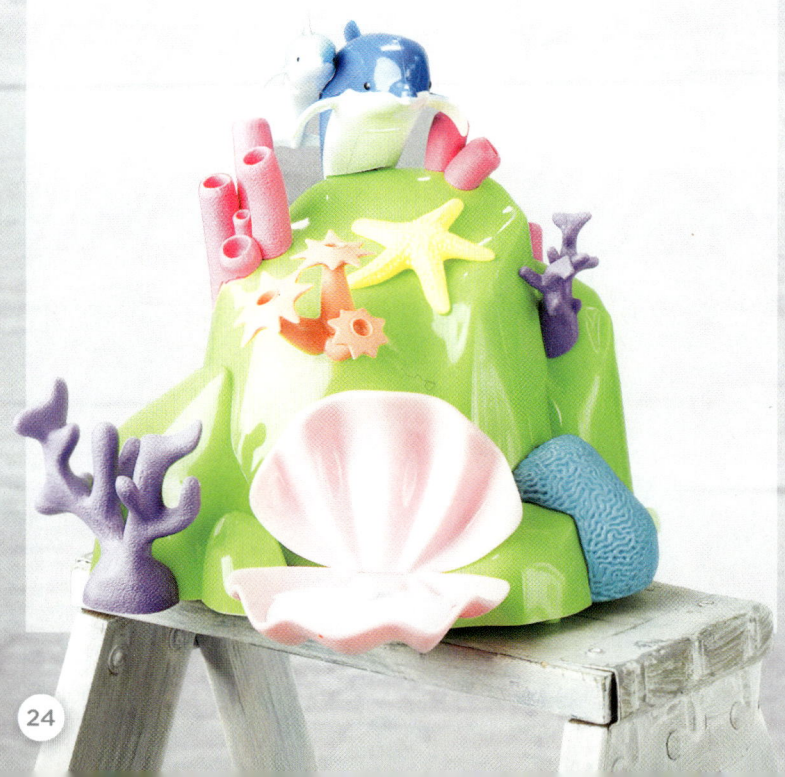

HOMEWORK HELPER

2 Drops Vetiver
2 Drops Lemon
2 Drops Cedarwood
3 Drops Clarity

TODDLER TIME

4 Drops Stress Away
3 Drops Citrus Fresh

YOU ARE MY SUNSHINE

2 Drops Orange
2 Drops Lemon
2 Drops Bergamot
2 Drops Lime
2 Drops Joy

STAND TALL

2 Drops Valor
2 Drops Envision
2 Drops Northern Lights Black Spruce

SWEET DREAMS

2 Drops Lavender
2 Drops Cedarwood
3 Drops Peace & Calming

BECAUSE IT'S NOT ALWAYS RAINBOWS & UNICORNS

One minute they are a princess without a care in the world, and the next minute they have transformed into the villain in your story. Children are often known to wear their emotions a little louder and more vibrant than their parents would choose. As you might imagine, there are oils that support happy moods. The basic citrus oils of Lemon, Lime, Orange, and Bergamot can quickly diffuse sour moods into sweet dispositions. On your quest to clean up the toxins in your home, you can start by removing all those synthetic plug-ins and candles and start diffusing these fresh scents, in classrooms, kitchens, bathrooms, bedrooms and anywhere your children play! Restore the Joy to your home and yes, you can create your own colorful rainbow at the end of your own story with Young Living essential oils!

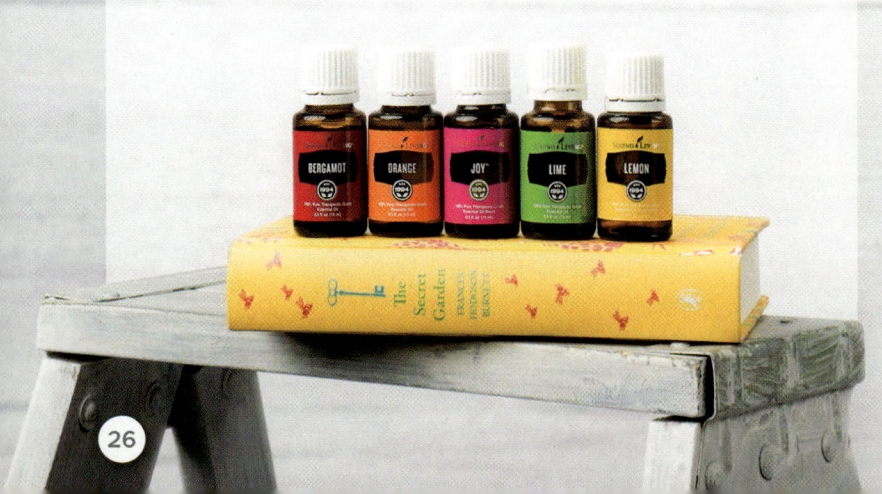

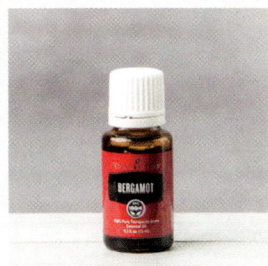

BERGAMOT

- Diffuse in your home or school classroom to jump start your day
- Add a drop to your child's favorite diffuser necklace

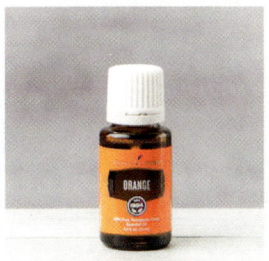

ORANGE

- Orange is an important ingredient in popular blends like Citrus Fresh, Christmas Spirit, and Peace & Calming
- Add 10 drops to a water spritz bottle to freshen your child's linens during the day

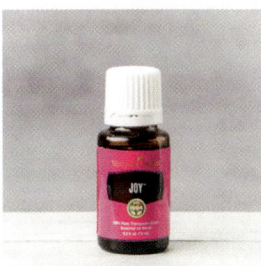

JOY™

- Blend of Bergamot, Ylang Ylang, Geranium, Lemon, Coriander, Tangerine, Jasmine, Roman Chamomile, Palmarosa, Rose essential oils
- Apply one drop over your child's heart before you send them off to school

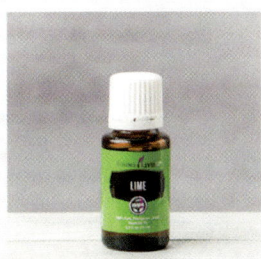

LIME

- Diffuse in the toddler's playroom
- Add a drop to your shampoo to rinse your Princess' scalp

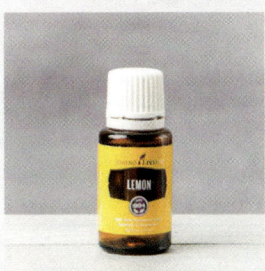

LEMON

- Add to a rag and clean your child's artwork off the walls and furniture
- Use a drop to take sticky sticker residue off toys

PAT-A-CAKE, BAKE ME A CAKE

Do you allow your little women and little men to help with meal time preparations? The healthy habits that are formed in childhood will carry over into adulthood. Kids love the hands-on bonding time spent with parents or grandparents in the kitchen helping prepare simple oil infused recipes. Did you know Young Living has an entire Vitality™ line of essential oils that can be added to your favorite recipes? These oils can add a splash of citrus to beverages, enhance the flavor of meats and veggies, and complement a sweet treat. Starting with these 5 vitality oils, you can make some Lavender shortbread cookies, Orange chicken, Lime salsa, Lemon cupcakes, or hot apple cider with a drop of Cinnamon Bark.

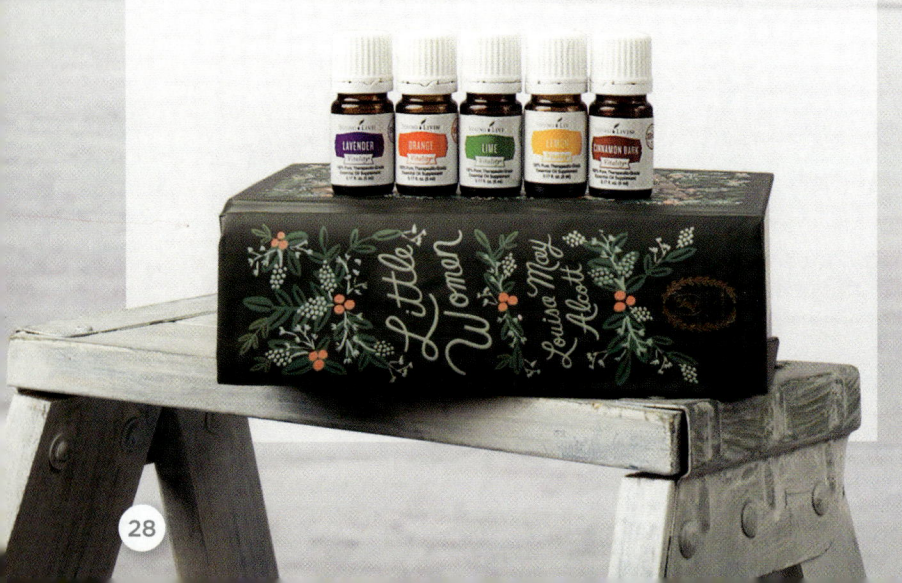

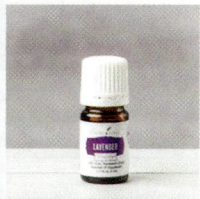

LAVENDER VITALITY™

- Make homemade jams and jellies infused with Lavender Vitality
- Great complement to homemade ice cream

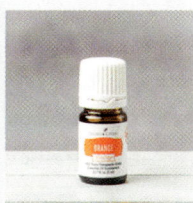

ORANGE VITALITY™

- Add a drop to your child's daily serving of NingXia Red®
- Mix with honey for an orange glaze on chicken nuggets

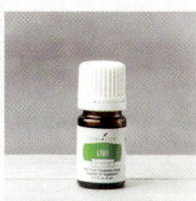

LIME VITALITY™

- Mix a few drops with honey and drizzle over a bowl of fresh fruit
- Add 3 drops to your homemade guacamole for little fingers to dip veggies in

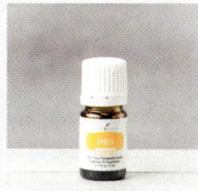

LEMON VITALITY™

- Add 5 drops to a lemon bar special treat
- Add 5 drops to a glass pitcher of homemade lemonade

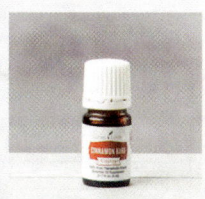

CINNAMON BARK VITALITY™

- Add 1 drop to a banana smoothie
- Add 1 drop to spice up a bowl of oatmeal or apple sauce

LAVENDER SHORTBREAD COOKIES

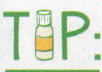

- 2 cups flour
- 1 cup cold butter, cubed
- 1/2 cup sugar
- 1/2 teaspoon salt
- 1 tablespoon water
- 1 teaspoon vanilla
- 5 drops Lavender Vitality

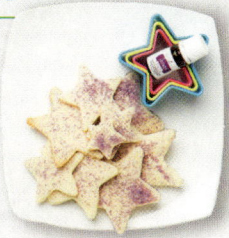

Mix all ingredients in mixer. Cover and refrigerate for 2 hours. Roll out dough on a flour covered surface. Cut with cookie cutter shape. Bake at 325° for 10 minutes.

YOUNG LIVING™
ESSENTIAL OILS

PREMIUM STARTER KIT
ALL ABOUT KIDS

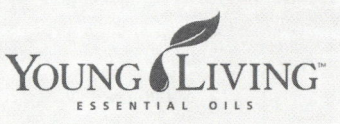

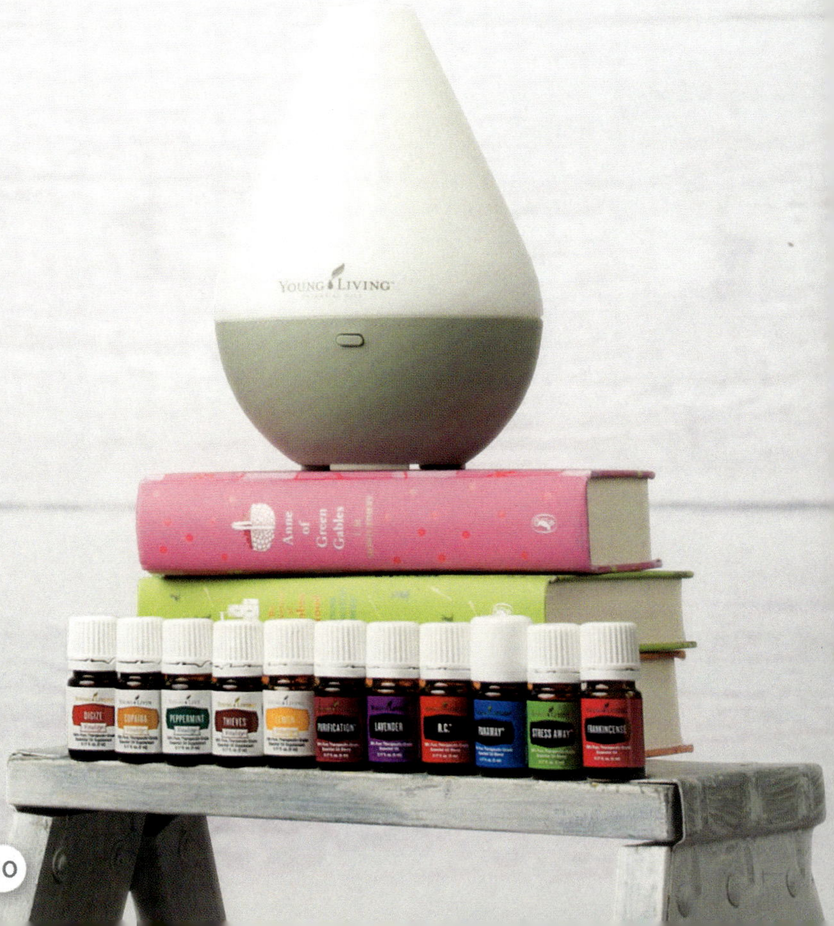

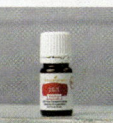
DIGIZE VITALITY™
- Add a drop to a spoon of honey before or after meals
- Add a drop to a glass of milk or almond milk before bedtime

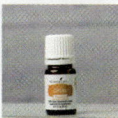
COPAIBA VITALITY™
- Add a drop to plain yogurt to promote and maintain wellness
- Add a drop to a frozen washcloth for teething toddlers to chew on

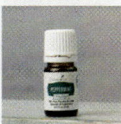
PEPPERMINT VITALITY™
- Add 5 drops to your brownie mix before baking
- Add 1 drop to a spoon of honey to support the digestive system

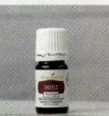
THIEVES VITALITY™
- Add a drop to homemade applesauce for a sweet treat
- Flavor homemade granola with a couple drops for a lunch box snack

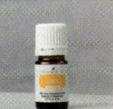
LEMON VITALITY™
- Add a couple drops to a pitcher of homemade lemonade
- Add 5 drops to your favorite lemon cookie recipe

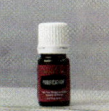
PURIFICATION®
- Add a drop to a cotton ball and place in stinky kid's shoes
- Boys! Enough said...Diffuse in bathrooms & neutralize sports equipment

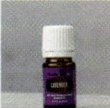
LAVENDER
- Add a drop to an Epsom salt bath and help kids unwind before bed
- Spritz your child's pillows before bed to promote relaxation

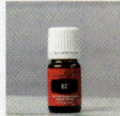
R.C.™
- Rub a drop with carrier oil on chest in the morning to promote a positive day
- Diffuse before bedtime

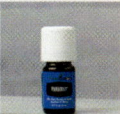
PANAWAY®
- Apply topically with coconut oil after sports activities
- For those clumsy moments

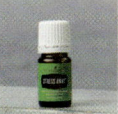
STRESS AWAY™
- Apply a drop on wrists in the morning before a test at school
- Sibling rivalry - Diffuse the situation with Stress Away

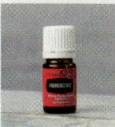
FRANKINCENSE
- Apply topically to children's skin to maintain its youthful appearance
- Diffuse to promote a peaceful environment for focus during study times

START SMART

All of the products we explored together are safe for 2-12 year olds, when used properly. It is always smart to start slowly with essential oils to allow body systems time to get used to something new. The KidScents® essential oils are formulated with this age group in mind and have been pre-diluted for easy application. On our journey we discussed 3 different ways to use essential oils:

Aromatically - smelling oils from bottle or diffusing

Topically - applying oils directly to skin

Internally - cooking; add to drinks or food to consume

Once you have decided you want to give essential oils a try, start by diffusing the oils in a home diffuser. This is a fantastic way to introduce your family to oils. Then move to diluting the oils with a carrier oil such as olive oil, coconut oil, or V-6™ enhanced vegetable oil complex and apply directly to the skin as suggested by directions on the bottle. A few essential oils like Peppermint and the Thieves® blend have a warming feel to them, so you will want to test those on a small area of skin or start by applying to the feet. The bottom of kid's feet are generally less sensitive, but also have contact points for the entire body. When you are feeling good about your family's response to aromatic and topical usage of essential oils, you can visit the white label Vitality oils and experiment with adding the essential oils to foods and beverages for your children and family to enjoy.